Care during Pregnancy

Farmina Taslim

Why I have Penned this Book

I have written the book *Care during Pregnancy* with the aim of providing comprehensive and reliable information to expectant mothers and their families. Pregnancy is a crucial period in a woman's life, and it is essential to ensure proper care and support throughout this journey. This book serves as a guide, offering valuable insights into various aspects of pregnancy, including physical and emotional changes, nutrition, exercise, prenatal care, common discomforts, and potential complications.

Furthermore, I felt compelled to write this book due to the lack of accessible and accurate resources on pregnancy care. Many women often find themselves overwhelmed by conflicting advice or unreliable sources of information. Therefore, my intention with *Care during Pregnancy* is to present evidence-based recommendations supported by medical professionals and experts in the field. By addressing common concerns and providing practical tips for a healthy pregnancy, I hope to empower women with knowledge that will enable them to make informed decisions about their own well-being and that of their unborn child.

In conclusion, my motivation for writing *Care during Pregnancy* stems from a genuine desire to contribute positively to the lives of expectant mothers by equipping them with reliable information and guidance. It is my hope that this book will serve as a trusted resource throughout their pregnancy journey, fostering confidence and promoting optimal health for both mother and baby.

Care during Pregnancy

Dedication

To my supporting husband Md. Ziaul Haque and our cute princess Azmiran Haq!

Contents

Chapter 1

The Beginnings of Care - Understanding Pregnancy

Introduction

Pregnancy, a miraculous journey of creation and life, is a time of profound changes, both physical and emotional, for the expectant mother. It marks the beginning of a new chapter, filled with excitement, joy, and perhaps some anxieties. The care provided during pregnancy plays a vital role in ensuring the health and well-being of both the mother and the unborn child. This book aims to guide you through the process of caring for yourself and your baby during this transformative period.

Section 1: The Wonders of Conception

The road to pregnancy begins with the fusion of an egg and a sperm, a process known as fertilization. This remarkable event typically occurs in the fallopian tubes after ovulation. Once fertilized, the egg starts dividing rapidly, forming a cluster of cells that gradually develop into an embryo.

As the embryo travels down the fallopian tube towards the uterus, it undergoes several stages of growth. By the time it reaches the uterus, it has become a blastocyst, consisting of two distinct cell types - the inner cell mass, which will become the baby, and the outer cells that will support its development.

Section 2: Understanding the Trimesters

Pregnancy is typically divided into three trimesters, each lasting approximately three months. During the first trimester, the baby's major organs and body systems begin to form, and the mother might experience morning sickness and fatigue as her body adapts to the changes.

In the second trimester, the baby's movements become noticeable, and the mother's belly starts to show. This is often considered the "golden period" of pregnancy, with many women feeling more energetic and experiencing a sense of well-being.

The third trimester brings the final stages of fetal development. The baby gains weight rapidly, and the mother may experience physical discomfort as the baby grows larger. Preparations for childbirth become a priority during this time.

Section 3: Prenatal Care - The Foundation of a Healthy Pregnancy

Prenatal care is the cornerstone of ensuring a healthy pregnancy. Regular check-ups with a healthcare provider are essential to monitor the mother's health and the baby's development. These visits typically include physical examinations, ultrasound scans, and various tests to assess the well-being of both the mother and the baby.

Nutrition during pregnancy is another crucial aspect of prenatal care. A well-balanced diet rich in essential nutrients supports the baby's growth and helps the mother maintain her own health. Special attention should be given to the intake of folic acid, iron, calcium, and other vitamins and minerals.

Section 4: Coping with Pregnancy Symptoms

Pregnancy brings about a myriad of physical and emotional changes that can vary from woman to woman. From morning sickness and heartburn to mood swings and fatigue, understanding and managing these symptoms can greatly improve the overall pregnancy experience.

Engaging in regular, moderate exercise can help alleviate discomfort and improve mood. Additionally, relaxation techniques, such as prenatal yoga and meditation, can help reduce stress and promote a sense of calmness.

Section 5: Preparing for Childbirth

As the pregnancy progresses, preparing for childbirth becomes a significant focus. Education about different birthing options, including natural childbirth, water births, and cesarean sections, allows expectant mothers to make informed decisions about their delivery.

Childbirth classes, both in-person and online, provide valuable information on labor, pain management techniques, and postpartum care. Partners can also participate in these classes, allowing them to offer support during labor and delivery.

Section 6: Emotional Well-being and Support

Pregnancy is not just a physical journey but an emotional one as well. Hormonal changes, coupled with the anticipation of becoming a parent, can lead to mood swings and feelings of anxiety. It is essential to prioritize emotional well-being and seek support from loved ones, friends, or even professional counselors if needed.

Conclusion

The first chapter of "Care During Pregnancy" has laid the foundation for understanding the incredible journey of pregnancy. From conception to childbirth, every step of this process deserves careful attention and care. Throughout this book, we will delve deeper into various aspects of pregnancy, exploring prenatal exercises, nutrition, labor and delivery, postpartum care, and much more. Remember, each pregnancy is unique, and embracing this beautiful experience with knowledge and preparation will ensure a healthy and fulfilling journey for both the mother and the baby.

Chapter 2

Nurturing a Healthy Pregnancy - Prenatal Nutrition and Exercise

Introduction

In Chapter 1, we explored the wonders of conception and the early stages of pregnancy. Now, as you progress through this miraculous journey, caring for your body and the growing life within it becomes paramount. In this chapter, we will focus on two fundamental aspects of prenatal care - nutrition and exercise. A well-balanced diet and regular physical activity are vital components of ensuring a healthy pregnancy and promoting the optimal development of your baby.

Section 1: Prenatal Nutrition - Fueling the Miracle

During pregnancy, your body undergoes remarkable changes to support the growth and development of your baby. Proper nutrition not only sustains your own health but also provides essential nutrients for the developing fetus. Let's explore the key components of a healthy prenatal diet:

1.1 Caloric Intake and Weight Gain

Pregnancy increases your caloric needs, but the idea that you need to "eat for two" is a myth. The additional calories required during pregnancy are relatively modest, especially during the first trimester. As a general guideline, most pregnant women need only about 300-500 extra calories per day in the second and third trimesters.

Healthy weight gain is a natural part of pregnancy, but it should be within a healthy range. Excessive weight gain can increase the risk of complications, while inadequate weight gain may lead to low birth weight. Your healthcare provider will monitor your weight and guide you on appropriate weight gain based on your individual circumstances.

1.2 Essential Nutrients

During pregnancy, certain nutrients are particularly crucial for both you and your baby's well-being:

1.2.1 Folic Acid: Folic acid is vital for early fetal development, particularly in preventing neural tube defects. Foods rich in folic acid include leafy greens, fortified cereals, and legumes. Many prenatal supplements also contain folic acid.

1.2.2 Iron: Iron is essential for producing hemoglobin, the protein in red blood cells that carries oxygen to cells throughout the body. Pregnant women need more iron to support the increased blood volume. Good sources of iron include lean meats, beans, tofu, and fortified cereals.

1.2.3 Calcium: Calcium is critical for the development of your baby's bones and teeth. Dairy products, fortified plant-based milk, and leafy greens are excellent sources of calcium.

1.2.4 Omega-3 Fatty Acids: Omega-3 fatty acids, particularly DHA, play a crucial role in the development of your baby's brain and eyes. Fatty fish like salmon, chia seeds, and walnuts are rich sources of omega-3s.

1.2.5 Vitamin D: Vitamin D is essential for bone health and may help prevent pregnancy complications. Sunlight is a natural source of vitamin D, and it can also be found in fortified dairy products and supplements.

1.3 Hydration

Staying well-hydrated is essential during pregnancy, as it helps maintain amniotic fluid levels and supports overall bodily functions. Aim to drink at least eight 8-ounce glasses of water daily, and more if you're physically active or during hot weather.

1.4 Foods to Avoid

Certain foods pose risks during pregnancy and should be avoided or limited. These include:

1.4.1 Raw or undercooked meats, eggs, and fish, which may carry harmful bacteria.

1.4.2 Unpasteurized dairy products and soft cheeses like brie and feta, as they may contain harmful bacteria.

1.4.3 High-mercury fish like shark, swordfish, and king mackerel, as mercury can harm the developing nervous system.

1.4.4 Caffeine and alcohol should be consumed in moderation or avoided altogether.

Section 2: Prenatal Exercise - Nurturing Your Body and Baby

Regular exercise during pregnancy can contribute to improved physical and emotional well-being for both you and your baby. However, it's essential to approach prenatal exercise with caution and choose activities that are safe and suitable for your changing body.

2.1 Benefits of Prenatal Exercise

Engaging in appropriate prenatal exercise offers numerous benefits, including:

2.1.1 Increased energy levels and reduced fatigue.

2.1.2 Improved posture and reduced back pain, common during pregnancy due to the growing belly.

2.1.3 Better sleep quality.

2.1.4 Enhanced mood and reduced risk of prenatal depression and anxiety.

2.1.5 Better physical stamina, which can be beneficial during labor and delivery.

2.2 Safe Prenatal Exercises

Not all exercises are suitable for pregnancy. It's essential to choose low-impact activities that reduce the risk of injury and strain on your body. Recommended prenatal exercises include:

2.2.1 Walking: A simple and effective way to stay active throughout pregnancy.

2.2.2 Swimming: Provides a full-body workout with minimal impact on joints.

2.2.3 Prenatal Yoga: Improves flexibility, strength, and relaxation. Focuses on breathing techniques beneficial during labor.

2.2.4 Low-impact Aerobics: Classes specifically designed for pregnant women, focusing on cardiovascular health.

2.2.5 Strength Training: Using light weights or resistance bands to maintain muscle tone and strength.

2.3 Activities to Avoid

Certain activities should be avoided during pregnancy, including:

2.3.1 High-impact sports with a high risk of falling or abdominal trauma.

2.3.2 Activities with a risk of overheating or dehydration.

2.3.3 Exercises that require lying flat on your back after the first trimester.

2.4 Listening to Your Body

As your body changes during pregnancy, it's essential to listen to its signals and modify your exercise routine accordingly. Avoid pushing yourself to the point of exhaustion, and always stay hydrated during physical activity.

Conclusion

In this chapter, we've explored the significance of prenatal nutrition and exercise in nurturing a healthy pregnancy. A well-balanced diet and regular physical activity lay the foundation for your baby's optimal development and your own well-being. Remember, each pregnancy is unique, and it's crucial to consult with your healthcare provider to develop a personalized plan that best suits your needs. In the next chapter, we will delve into the various prenatal screening and diagnostic tests, providing insights into their importance and how they can aid in ensuring a healthy pregnancy.

<u>Chapter 3</u>

Ensuring a Healthy Pregnancy - Prenatal Screening and Diagnostic Tests

Introduction

As you embark on the journey of pregnancy, your healthcare provider will recommend a series of prenatal screening and diagnostic tests. These tests are designed to assess the health and development of both you and your baby. In Chapter 3, we will explore the various prenatal tests available, their significance, and how they contribute to ensuring a healthy pregnancy.

Section 1: Prenatal Screening Tests

Prenatal screening tests are non-invasive procedures that assess the risk of certain genetic conditions and birth defects. These tests do not provide definitive answers but help identify individuals who may require further diagnostic testing.

1.1 First Trimester Screening

First-trimester screening is typically conducted between weeks 10 and 13 of pregnancy and consists of two components:

1.1.1 Nuchal Translucency (NT) Test: This ultrasound measurement assesses the thickness of the fluid at the back of the baby's neck. An increased NT measurement may indicate a higher risk of certain chromosomal abnormalities.

1.1.2 Blood Test: The blood test measures specific proteins and hormones in the mother's blood. Combined with the NT measurement and other factors such as maternal age, it provides an estimate of the risk of conditions like Down syndrome and trisomy 18.

1.2 Cell-Free DNA Testing (cfDNA)

Cell-free DNA testing, also known as non-invasive prenatal testing (NIPT), is a blood test that analyzes fetal DNA circulating in the mother's bloodstream. This test is typically conducted after the first-trimester screening and is particularly effective at detecting certain chromosomal conditions, such as Down syndrome, with a high degree of accuracy.

1.3 Quad Screen (Second-Trimester Screening)

The quad screen, also known as the quadruple marker test, is performed between weeks 15 and 20 of pregnancy. This blood test measures four substances in the mother's blood - alpha-fetoprotein (AFP), human chorionic gonadotropin (hCG), estriol, and inhibin A. The quad screen assesses the risk of neural tube defects and chromosomal conditions.

Section 2: Prenatal Diagnostic Tests

Unlike screening tests, prenatal diagnostic tests provide definitive answers regarding the presence or absence of certain genetic conditions and birth defects. However, they are invasive and carry a small risk of miscarriage.

2.1 Chorionic Villus Sampling (CVS)

Chorionic villus sampling is usually performed between weeks 10 and 13 of pregnancy. During the procedure, a small sample of tissue (chorionic villi) is taken from the placenta and analyzed for genetic abnormalities. CVS can diagnose chromosomal conditions and some genetic disorders.

2.2 Amniocentesis

Amniocentesis is typically performed between weeks 15 and 20 of pregnancy. A thin needle is inserted through the abdomen into the amniotic sac to collect a sample of amniotic fluid. This fluid contains fetal cells that can be analyzed for chromosomal abnormalities and genetic disorders.

2.3 Diagnostic Ultrasound

Diagnostic ultrasounds are non-invasive imaging tests that use sound waves to create pictures of the baby and the uterus. These ultrasounds can provide valuable information about the baby's growth and development, detect multiple pregnancies, and identify structural abnormalities.

Section 3: Prenatal Testing for Gestational Diabetes and Group B Streptococcus (GBS)

3.1 Gestational Diabetes Screening

Gestational diabetes is a form of diabetes that develops during pregnancy and can affect both the mother and the baby's health. Typically, between weeks 24 and 28 of pregnancy, a glucose challenge test is performed. If the initial screening indicates elevated blood sugar levels, a glucose tolerance test may be conducted to confirm the diagnosis.

3.2 Group B Streptococcus (GBS) Screening

Group B Streptococcus is a type of bacteria that can be present in the vagina or rectum of some pregnant women. While it usually doesn't cause issues for the mother, it can be transmitted to the baby during childbirth and lead to serious infections. GBS screening is typically performed between weeks 35 and 37 of pregnancy. If GBS is detected, antibiotics can be administered during labor to reduce the risk of transmission to the baby.

Section 4: Understanding Test Results and Making Informed Decisions

Receiving the results of prenatal tests can be an emotional and challenging experience. It's crucial to remember that these tests are meant to provide information, not predictions. Abnormal results do not guarantee that a baby will have a specific condition, and normal results do not guarantee a completely healthy baby.

It's essential to discuss test results with your healthcare provider thoroughly. They will help you understand the implications and guide you through the decision-making process if further testing or interventions are necessary.

Conclusion

Chapter 3 has provided an overview of prenatal screening and diagnostic tests. These tests play a vital role in assessing the health and development of both the mother and the baby. Prenatal care involves a comprehensive approach that includes monitoring nutrition, exercise, and screening for potential health concerns. By working closely with your healthcare provider and making informed decisions, you can ensure the best possible care for yourself and your baby throughout this transformative journey of pregnancy. In the next chapter, we will delve into the physical and emotional changes that occur during the second trimester and explore strategies to cope with them effectively.

Chapter 4

Embracing the Second Trimester - Coping with Physical and Emotional Changes

Introduction

As you enter the second trimester of pregnancy, you may find yourself feeling more settled and energized. The second trimester, often referred to as the "golden period" of pregnancy, spans from weeks 13 to 28. During this time, many women experience relief from early pregnancy symptoms and a renewed sense of well-being. However, the second trimester also brings its own set of physical and emotional changes that warrant attention and care. In this chapter, we will explore the unique aspects of the second trimester and strategies to cope with them effectively.

Section 1: Physical Changes and Their Management

1.1 Growing Belly and Weight Gain

As your baby continues to grow, your belly will become more noticeable, and weight gain will likely accelerate. Embrace your changing body, as this is a natural and beautiful part of pregnancy. However, it's essential to maintain a healthy weight gain, as excessive weight gain can lead to complications such as gestational diabetes and high blood pressure.

- Follow your healthcare provider's guidance on weight gain during pregnancy.
- Continue to eat a well-balanced diet rich in essential nutrients.
- Engage in regular, safe physical activity to support your overall health and manage weight.

1.2 Stretch Marks

Stretch marks are common during pregnancy and can appear on your belly, breasts, hips, and thighs as your skin stretches to accommodate your growing baby. While it may not be possible to prevent stretch marks entirely, keeping your skin moisturized and hydrated can help reduce their severity.

- Use a gentle, hypoallergenic moisturizer to keep your skin hydrated.
- Massage your skin regularly to improve circulation and elasticity.

1.3 Back Pain and Body Aches

As your baby grows and your center of gravity shifts, you may experience back pain and body aches, particularly in the lower back. Hormonal changes can also contribute to joint laxity, leading to discomfort.

- Practice good posture and use supportive pillows while sitting and sleeping.

- Engage in prenatal exercises, such as yoga and swimming, to strengthen your core and alleviate back pain.
- Seek prenatal massage or physical therapy if needed.

1.4 Varicose Veins and Swollen Feet

Increased blood volume during pregnancy can lead to varicose veins, which are swollen and twisted veins, often found in the legs. Additionally, fluid retention may cause swelling in your feet and ankles.

- Avoid prolonged periods of standing or sitting; take breaks to elevate your legs.
- Wear comfortable, supportive shoes that allow for proper circulation.
- Compression stockings can help alleviate varicose vein discomfort.

Section 2: Coping with Emotional Changes

2.1 Bonding with Your Baby

During the second trimester, you may start feeling your baby's movements, also known as quickening. This can be a magical experience that fosters a sense of connection between you and your little one.

- Take time each day to focus on your baby and communicate with them through gentle touches and talking.

- Involve your partner and loved ones in the process, sharing the joy of feeling the baby's kicks.

2.2 Managing Mood Swings

Pregnancy hormones can lead to mood swings, causing you to feel elated one moment and teary-eyed the next.

- Engage in activities that promote relaxation, such as prenatal yoga and meditation.
- Talk openly with your partner and support network about your emotions and seek understanding and comfort when needed.

2.3 Addressing Anxiety and Fears

As your pregnancy progresses, you may develop anxieties and fears about childbirth and becoming a parent. These emotions are entirely normal and shared by many expectant mothers.

- Attend childbirth education classes to learn about the birthing process and ease fears surrounding labor.
- Discuss your concerns with your healthcare provider, who can provide reassurance and address any questions.

Section 3: Bonding with Your Partner

The second trimester can be an ideal time to strengthen the bond with your partner as you both prepare for parenthood.

- Attend prenatal appointments together to share the excitement of seeing ultrasound images and hearing your baby's heartbeat.
- Engage in activities that promote relaxation and connection, such as taking walks, reading to your baby, or creating a baby journal together.

Conclusion

In this chapter, we've explored the physical and emotional changes that occur during the second trimester of pregnancy. As you continue on this extraordinary journey, remember to care for your changing body and nurture your emotional well-being. Embrace the joys of feeling your baby move and cherish the moments of connection with your partner. By acknowledging and addressing the challenges and changes of the second trimester, you can make the most of this special time as you prepare to welcome your little one into the world. In the next chapter, we will delve into the preparations for childbirth and explore various birthing options to help you make informed decisions for your delivery experience.

Chapter 5

A Joyful Arrival - Preparing for Childbirth and Postpartum Care

Introduction

As you approach the final weeks of pregnancy, the excitement and anticipation of meeting your baby grow exponentially. The moment of childbirth marks the culmination of this incredible journey, bringing forth new life and parenthood. In this final chapter, we will explore the preparations for childbirth, the various birthing options available, and the essential aspects of postpartum care to ensure a smooth transition into motherhood.

Section 1: Preparing for Childbirth

1.1 Childbirth Education Classes

Childbirth education classes are an invaluable resource for expectant parents, providing essential information and tools for labor and delivery. These classes cover topics such as the stages of labor, pain management techniques, and postpartum care.

- Enroll in childbirth education classes early in the third trimester to allow ample time for learning and practice.
- Attend classes with your partner or support person to share knowledge and support each other during labor.

1.2 Creating a Birth Plan

A birth plan outlines your preferences and desires for labor and delivery. While it's essential to remain flexible, a birth plan can help you communicate your preferences to your healthcare providers and ensure your wishes are respected, to the extent possible.

- Discuss your birth plan with your healthcare provider and address any questions or concerns they may have.
- Be prepared for unexpected changes in the birth plan and trust your medical team's expertise.

1.3 Packing Your Hospital Bag

As your due date approaches, it's essential to have a hospital bag packed and ready to go. Include essential items such as comfortable clothing, toiletries, snacks, and items for your baby, like clothes and blankets.

- Keep important documents, such as identification and insurance information, in your bag.
- Consider including items that provide comfort and relaxation, such as your favorite pillow or music.

Section 2: Birthing Options

2.1 Vaginal Birth

Vaginal birth is the most common method of childbirth, where the baby is born through the birth canal. It can be a natural birth or may involve pain management techniques, such as epidurals or nitrous oxide, to manage discomfort.

- Attend childbirth education classes to learn about the stages of labor and various coping techniques for a vaginal birth.
- Discuss your preferences for pain management with your healthcare provider.

2.2 Cesarean Section (C-Section)

A cesarean section is a surgical procedure in which the baby is delivered through an incision in the abdomen and uterus. C-sections may be planned in advance or performed in emergencies.

- Learn about the circumstances that may necessitate a C-section and discuss any concerns with your healthcare provider.
- Prepare for post-operative recovery following a C-section.

2.3 Water Birth

Water birth involves giving birth in a pool or tub of warm water. Some women find water birth to be soothing and empowering during labor.

- Discuss the possibility of a water birth with your healthcare provider and inquire about water birthing facilities at your chosen birthing center or hospital.

- Ensure the water temperature remains at a safe and comfortable level for both you and the baby.

Section 3: Postpartum Care

3.1 Immediate Postpartum Period

The immediate postpartum period, often referred to as the "golden hour," is a critical time for bonding with your baby and initiating breastfeeding if desired. Your healthcare provider and support team will monitor you and your baby's well-being during this time.

- Take advantage of skin-to-skin contact with your baby, as it helps regulate their body temperature and fosters bonding.
- Seek support from lactation consultants or nurses if you choose to breastfeed.

3.2 Emotional Well-being

The postpartum period can bring a range of emotions, from joy and elation to exhaustion and feelings of overwhelm.

- Communicate openly with your partner and loved ones about your emotional experiences.
- Seek help and support if you experience symptoms of postpartum depression or anxiety.

3.3 Physical Recovery

Postpartum recovery involves allowing your body time to heal after childbirth.

- Rest as much as possible and avoid strenuous activities during the initial weeks postpartum.
- Follow your healthcare provider's guidance on wound care (if applicable) and postpartum exercise.

3.4 Bonding with Your Baby

The postpartum period presents opportunities for deepening the bond with your baby.

- Engage in frequent skin-to-skin contact and gentle touch to promote bonding.
- Participate in feeding and diaper-changing routines to connect with your baby.

Conclusion

As you prepare to welcome your baby into the world, remember that childbirth is a unique and transformative experience. Embrace the uncertainty and embrace the joy of meeting your little one for the first time. By being informed, prepared, and open to the journey ahead, you can approach childbirth and postpartum care with confidence and grace. Embrace the support of your healthcare team, partner, and loved ones as you navigate the challenges and rewards of motherhood. Cherish each moment and celebrate the miracle of new life, knowing that you are equipped with the knowledge and tools to provide the best possible care for yourself and your baby. Congratulations on this new chapter in your life - welcome to the beautiful world of motherhood.

About the Author

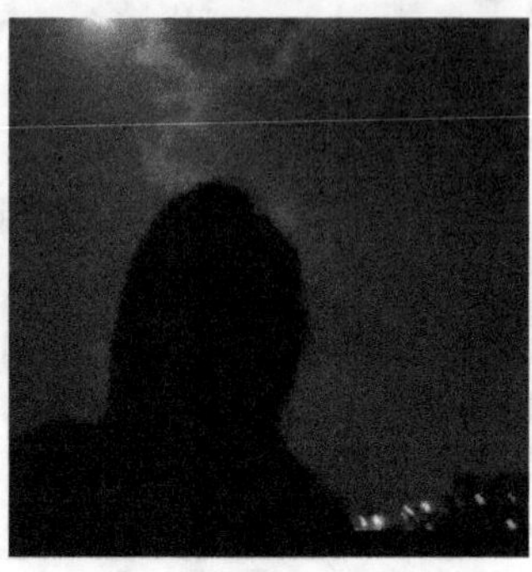

Farmina Taslim is a dynamic and versatile professional with a passion for storytelling and a gift for words. She possesses a Master's in Sociology from Dhaka University, Bangladesh. With a background in journalism and a flair for writing, she has established herself as a skilled journalist and writer. Her ability to conduct thorough research, ask thought-provoking questions, and craft engaging narratives has earned her recognition in the field. Whether it is covering breaking news, exploring human interest stories, or delving into cultural phenomena, Farmina's dedication to providing accurate and captivating content shines through in her work.

In addition to her prowess as a journalist and writer, Farmina is a proficient vlogger and content creator. With her creative vision and natural on-camera presence, she captivates audiences through her informative and entertaining videos. Her ability to adapt her storytelling skills to different mediums allows her to engage viewers and readers alike, bringing stories to life in engaging and accessible ways. Beyond creating content, Farmina's attention to detail and language expertise serve her well as an editor, proofreader, and translator. Her meticulous approach ensures that written materials are polished to perfection and effectively convey their intended messages across various languages and cultural contexts. Farmina's versatile skill set and commitment to producing high-quality content make her an invaluable asset in the media industry and also in the world of literature.

List of Her Books

Short Story:

1. The Mysterious Case [2023]

2. A Serial Killer [2023]

3. Stories of Diaspora [2023]

4. Lost Treasure [2023]

5. Psychological Thrillers [2023]

6. Women's Crime Fiction [2023]

7. Hidden Truth [2023]

8. Horror Stories [2023]

Non-fiction:

1. 150 Facts about Your Wife [2023]

2. 200 Facts about Your Husband [2023]

3. Care before Pregnancy [2023]

Farmina Taslim

E-mail

farminatasliim@gmail.com

Twitter

https://twitter.com/Farmina_Taslim?t=eQcvL-

5op1ZRC24TfxCu1g&s=09

Facebook

https://www.facebook.com/farmina.taslim?mibextid=Zb

WKwL

Instagram

https://instagram.com/farmina_taslim?igshid=NTc4MTI

wNjQ2YQ==

YouTube

https://www.youtube.com/channel/UCmvjdHLbQ-

W7OSX8p-MiIkg

LinkedIn

https://www.linkedin.com/in/farmina-taslim-86b432190

TikTok

https://www.tiktok.com/@farminataslim?_t=8dAXqyUVP

eC&_r=1